Healthy life for working women

By

James Vince

Table of content

Introduction 1

Chapter 1 3

Balancing Act: Juggling Work and Well-being.................3

Understanding the Dilemma.....................................3

The Holistic Approach to Work-Life Balance 4

Setting Boundaries:...4

Prioritizing Self-Care: 5

Effective Time Management:.....................................5

Embracing Flexibility: 5

Cultivating Emotional Intelligence: 6

The Psychological Impact of Imbalance 6

The Strain of Unrealistic Expectations: 6

The Vicious Cycle of Guilt:..7

Impact on Mental Health:...7

Strained Relationships: 7

Strategies for Success 8

Clarifying Personal Values:..8

Goal Setting with Purpose: 8

Seeking Support:...8

Embracing Continuous Learning: 9

Cultivating Mindfulness: 9

Empowering Others:..9

Embracing Imperfection: 10

Conclusion..10

Chapter 2 11

Nourishing Your Body and Mind Amidst the Hustle 11

Introduction: 11

The Neglected Foundations: Nutrition and Hydration
....11

Fueling Your Body: 12

Hydration as a Cornerstone: 12

Mindful Eating in a Fast-Paced World.....................12

Breaking Free from Multitasking: 13

Understanding Hunger and Fullness:......................13

Choosing Quality Over Quantity: 13

Cultivating Mental Nourishment: Strategies for Mind
Wellness...14

Moments of Mindfulness:........................14

Strategic Breaks for Mental Renewal: 14

Digital Detox for Mental Clarity: 15

Cultivating a Growth Mindset:................15

Connecting with Passions: 15

Physical Activity: A Pillar of Well-being.................16

Incorporating Movement into Daily Life:..............16

Choosing Activities, You Enjoy: 16

Prioritizing Consistency Over Intensity: 17

Strategies for Implementation: Turning Intentions
into Action 17

Creating a Well-being Plan:...................17

Scheduling Self-Care Time: 18

Building a Support System: 18

Adapting to Change: 18

Celebrating Small Wins:.....................................18

Conclusion: Thriving Amidst the Hustle 19

Chapter 3 20

Crafting a Sustainable Work-Life Harmony.................20

Introduction: 20

Redefining Work-Life Harmony 20

Shift from Balance to Harmony: 20

The Myth of Perfect Balance: 21

Elements of Sustainable Work-Life Harmony 21

Clarifying Priorities:...21

Defining Success on Your Terms: 21

Establishing Boundaries:.....................................22

Embracing Flexibility: 22

Mindful Time Management: 22

Investing in Self-Care: 23

Cultivating Interpersonal Relationships:...................23

Continuous Learning and Growth:..........................23

Navigating Challenges:..24

Overcoming Guilt and Expectations: 24

Communication and Advocacy: 24

Managing Burnout:..24

Technology and Disconnecting: 25

Success Stories and Inspirations: 25

Company Culture that Values Harmony: 25

Individuals Who Have Mastered Harmony: 25

Conclusion: A Lifelong Journey 26

Chapter 4 27

The Power of Mindfulness: Stress Management
Techniques..27

Understanding Mindfulness: 27

A Present-Moment Focus: 27

Mindfulness Meditation: 28

Bringing Mindfulness into Daily Life: 28

The Science Behind Mindfulness and Stress
Reduction:..28

Impact on the Brain: 28

Cortisol Regulation: 29

Enhanced Emotional Regulation:...............29

Mindfulness-Based Stress Reduction (MBSR):..........29

Structured Programs for Stress Reduction: 29

Components of MBSR:..............................30

Mindfulness in the Workplace:..................30

Enhancing Focus and Productivity: 30

Stress Reduction in Corporate Settings: 30

Practical Mindfulness Techniques for Stress
Management: 31

Mindful Breathing:..................................31

Body Scan Meditation:.............................31

Mindful Walking: 32

Mindful Eating: 32

Mindful Technology Use: 32

Challenges and Misconceptions: 33

Patience and Consistency: 33

Misconceptions about Mindfulness:.....................33

Cultivating a Mindful Lifestyle: 33

Mindful Communication: 33

Gratitude Practices: 34

Conclusion: Empowerment through Mindfulness 34

Chapter 5 36

Fitness on the Fly: Quick Workouts for Busy Schedules
....36

The Significance of Physical Activity: 36

Beyond Aesthetics: 36

Stress Reduction: 37

Boosting Productivity:..37

The Fitness on the Fly Approach:...................................37

Short Bursts of Activity: 37

Minimal Equipment: 38

Adaptability to Any Setting:....................................38

Quick Workouts for Busy Schedules: 38

High-Intensity Interval Training (HIIT):......................39

Tabata Training: 39

Bodyweight Circuits: 39

Quick Cardio Blasts: 40

Power Yoga or Pilates: 40

Resistance Band Exercises: 40

Quick Core Workouts:..40

Strategies for Incorporating Fitness on the Fly:............41

Schedule It: 41

Make It a Habit: 41

Maximize Breaks: 42

Utilize Technology:..42

Combine Activities: 42

Overcoming Common Challenges:..............................42

Overcoming Perfectionism: 42

Creating a Supportive Environment:.......................43

Prioritizing Self-Care: 43

Conclusion: 43

Chapter 6 45

Mindful Eating Strategies for Busy Professionals:
Nourishing Your Body and Mind in the Midst of Chaos45

Introduction: 45

The Importance of Mindful Eating:........................45

Benefits of Mindful Eating for Busy Professionals: 46

Improved Digestion: 46

Weight Management:..46

Stress Reduction: 47

Increased Energy Levels:....................................47

Enhanced Focus and Productivity: 47

Practical Mindful Eating Strategies for Busy
Professionals:...47

Set aside dedicated meal times: 47

Minimize distractions: 48

Practice gratitude before meals: 48

Chew slowly and savor each bite: 48

Listen to your body's signals: 48

Choose nutrient-dense foods: 49

Plan and prepare meals in advance: 49

Practice mindful breathing: 49

Create mindful eating rituals: 49

Stay flexible and be forgiving: 50

Conclusion: 50

Chapter 7 51

Building Resilience: A Comprehensive Guide to Coping with Workplace Challenges 51

Introduction: 51

The Importance of Resilience in the Workplace: 51

Adaptability to Change: 52

Stress Management: 52

Enhanced Problem-Solving: 52

Positive Work Relationships: 52

Increased Productivity: 53

Common Workplace Challenges: 53

High Workload and Tight Deadlines: 53

Interpersonal Conflicts: 53

Job Insecurity: 53

Lack of Recognition: 54

Organizational Changes: 54

Work-Life Imbalance:..54

Building and Enhancing Resilience:.....................................54

Cultivate a Growth Mindset:...55

Set Realistic Goals:..55

Prioritize Self-Care:...55

Seek Professional Development:..55

Maintain a Positive Mindset:...56

Build a Support System:...56

Develop Problem-Solving Skills:...56

Foster Flexibility:...56

Set Boundaries:..56

Conclusion:..57

Chapter 8 58

Sleep Smart: The Foundation of a Productive Day 58

Introduction:..58

Understanding the Importance of Quality Sleep:.........58

Physical Restoration:..58

Cognitive Function:..59

Emotional Well-being:...59

Metabolic Balance:..59

Cardiovascular Health:..59

The Impact of Sleep on Productivity:............................60

Enhanced Cognitive Performance:.......................................60

Increased Efficiency:..60

Better Decision-Making:..60

Effective Stress Management:..61

Improved Interpersonal Skills: 61

Practical Strategies for Smart Sleep:.........................61

Establish a Consistent Sleep Schedule: 61

Create a Relaxing Bedtime Routine: 61

Optimize Your Sleep Environment:............................62

Limit Exposure to Screens Before Bed: 62

Mind Your Diet:...62

Get Regular Exercise: 62

Manage Stress and Anxiety:.....................................63

Limit Naps: 63

Invest in Quality Sleepwear: 63

Seek Professional Help if Needed: 63

Conclusion: 63

Chapter 9 65

Navigating Social and Professional Networks with Grace: Building Meaningful Connections for Success 65

Introduction: 65

The Importance of Social and Professional Networks: .66

Opportunities for Growth: 66

Knowledge Exchange: 66

Support System:...66

Career Advancement: 67

Enhanced Visibility:..67

Challenges Associated with Networking:.....................67

Authenticity vs. Image Management:..........................67

Navigating Power Dynamics: 67

Building Meaningful Connections: 68

Overcoming Introversion: 68

Maintaining Balance: 68

Practical Strategies for Navigating Networks with Grace: 68

Be Authentic: 68

Active Listening: 69

Find Common Ground: 69

Effective Communication: 69

Navigate Power Dynamics with Sensitivity: 69

Cultivate a Diverse Network: 70

Set Realistic Networking Goals: 70

Utilize Online Platforms Wisely: 70

Follow Up and Stay Connected: 70

Build a Support System: 70

Invest in Personal Development: 71

Balance Quantity and Quality: 71

Conclusion: 71

Chapter 10 73

Cultivating Joy: Finding Happiness in Everyday Moments 73

Introduction: 73

Gratitude and Appreciation: 73

Enhanced Mental Well-being: 73

Positive Perspective: 74

Resilience in Adversity: 74

Connection and Relationships: 74

Psychological Benefits of Cultivating Joy: 75

Stress Reduction: 75

Improved Mood and Emotional Resilience:..............75

Increased Life Satisfaction: 75

Boosted Creativity and Productivity: 75

Better Physical Health:..76

Practical Strategies for Cultivating Joy in Everyday
Moments: 76

Practice Mindfulness: 76

Keep a Gratitude Journal: 76

Celebrate Small Achievements: 77

Create Rituals and Traditions:.................................77

Surround Yourself with Positivity: 77

Engage in Hobbies: 77

Express Gratitude to Others: 77

Find Joy in Nature: 78

Practice Positive Self-Talk: 78

Cultivate a positive inner dialogue. 78

Limit Screen Time: 78

Embrace the Power of Laughter: 78

Learn from Children:...79

Conclusion: 79

Introduction

In the fast-paced and demanding landscape of today's professional world, women are often confronted with the intricate task of balancing career aspirations with personal well-being. "Healthy Life for Working Women" is a guide tailored to address the unique challenges faced by women in the workforce, offering a holistic approach to foster physical, mental, and emotional vitality.

As women continue to make significant strides in diverse fields, the need for a comprehensive guide to maintaining a healthy lifestyle has become increasingly crucial. This book aims to empower working women with practical insights and actionable strategies, acknowledging the intricate dance between professional responsibilities and personal health.

From navigating stress and achieving work-life harmony to incorporating quick yet effective workouts into busy schedules, each chapter is designed to cater to the multifaceted dimensions of a woman's life. Mindful eating, resilience building, and the importance of quality sleep are explored as essential components of overall well-being. Through these pages, readers will discover how to not only survive but thrive in the challenging world of work, fostering a sustainable and fulfilling life that goes beyond the confines of the professional sphere.

"Healthy Life for Working Women" is a beacon of support and guidance for women seeking to navigate the intricacies of modern work environments while prioritizing their health and happiness.

Chapter 1

Balancing Act: Juggling Work and Well-being

In the relentless rhythm of the modern workplace, where deadlines loom and responsibilities multiply, finding equilibrium between career ambitions and personal well-being becomes a formidable challenge, particularly for working women. The delicate art of balancing work and well-being requires a strategic approach that considers the multifaceted dimensions of life, encompassing physical health, mental resilience, and emotional fulfillment.

Understanding the Dilemma

The contemporary professional landscape demands more from individuals than ever before. For working women, the challenge is twofold, as societal expectations and personal aspirations intertwine. The pressing need to break through glass ceilings, coupled with the traditional expectations placed on women in terms of caregiving and nurturing roles, creates a complex tapestry of responsibilities. The result is a perpetual juggling act that often leaves little room for self-care.

This balancing act is not merely about managing a to-do list or calendar; it's about reconciling the demands of the workplace with the need for personal sustenance. It involves acknowledging the interconnectedness of professional and personal spheres and recognizing that neglecting one invariably affects the other. Striking this delicate balance is not only crucial for individual well-being but also for sustained professional success.

The Holistic Approach to Work-Life Balance

Achieving a harmonious work-life balance is not a one-size-fits-all endeavor. It requires a holistic approach that considers the unique circumstances and aspirations of each individual. Recognizing the symbiotic relationship between work and personal life is the first step in this journey.

Setting Boundaries:

Establishing clear boundaries is fundamental to maintaining balance. This involves delineating specific times for work and personal life, creating a structured routine that accommodates both professional and personal priorities. Setting realistic expectations for oneself and communicating these boundaries with colleagues fosters a supportive work environment.

Prioritizing Self-Care:

In the relentless pursuit of career goals, self-care often takes a backseat. However, prioritizing physical and mental well-being is not a luxury but a necessity. This includes regular exercise, sufficient sleep, and mindful practices such as meditation. Recognizing the importance of self-care as an integral part of the work-life equation is essential for long-term success.

Effective Time Management:

Time is a finite resource, and mastering its management is key to achieving balance. Implementing effective time management techniques, such as the Pomodoro Technique or the Eisenhower Matrix, can enhance productivity and create space for personal pursuits. It's not about doing more but doing what matters most efficiently.

Embracing Flexibility:

Flexibility is a cornerstone of modern work environments, and embracing it can be instrumental in achieving work-life balance. Negotiating flexible work hours or remote work options, when feasible, provides the freedom to adapt schedules to personal needs. This flexibility fosters a sense of autonomy and control over one's professional and personal life.

Cultivating Emotional Intelligence:

Emotional intelligence is paramount in navigating the complexities of professional and personal relationships. Being attuned to one's own emotions and those of others allows for better communication, conflict resolution, and collaboration. This, in turn, contributes to a positive work environment and a more fulfilling personal life.

The Psychological Impact of Imbalance

The consequences of an imbalance between work and well-being are not confined to physical exhaustion; they extend to the realm of mental health. Burnout, a pervasive issue in high-pressure work environments, can manifest as chronic stress, emotional fatigue, and a sense of disillusionment. Working women, already grappling with societal expectations and gender biases, are particularly susceptible to the psychological toll of imbalance.

The Strain of Unrealistic Expectations:

Society's expectations of women often include the ability to effortlessly manage both professional and personal realms. This unrealistic ideal places undue pressure on working women, fostering a sense of inadequacy when confronted with the inevitable challenges of balancing work and well-being.

The Vicious Cycle of Guilt:

Juggling numerous responsibilities can evoke feelings of guilt when dedicating time to one aspect of life seemingly at the expense of another. The guilt associated with not meeting perceived expectations, whether at work or in personal life, creates a vicious cycle that undermines well-being and exacerbates the struggle for balance.

Impact on Mental Health:

Prolonged imbalance can take a toll on mental health, leading to conditions such as anxiety and depression. The relentless pursuit of professional success without adequate self-care amplifies stressors, contributing to a decline in mental well-being. Recognizing the signs of mental distress and seeking support are vital steps in mitigating these effects.

Strained Relationships:

The ripple effect of imbalance extends to personal relationships, with partners, children, and extended family members often bearing the brunt of unmet emotional needs. Strained relationships at home can, in turn, exacerbate stress in the workplace, creating a cyclical pattern of discontent.

Strategies for Success

Achieving a sustainable balance between work and well-being requires intentional effort and a commitment to self-discovery. Implementing strategies that align with individual values and priorities is key to navigating this delicate equilibrium.

Clarifying Personal Values:

Understanding one's core values is essential in making decisions that align with personal priorities. This clarity serves as a compass in navigating the myriad choices presented in both professional and personal spheres.

Goal Setting with Purpose:

Setting realistic and purpose-driven goals provides direction and motivation. These goals should encompass both professional aspirations and personal fulfillment, ensuring a holistic approach to success.

Seeking Support:

Recognizing the need for support is a strength, not a weakness. Seeking mentorship, building a support network, and fostering open communication with colleagues and family members create a foundation for navigating challenges with resilience.

Embracing Continuous Learning:

The dynamic nature of both the professional and personal realms necessitates a commitment to continuous learning. Adapting to new challenges and acquiring new skills not only enhances professional growth but also contributes to a sense of personal fulfillment.

Cultivating Mindfulness:

Mindfulness, the practice of being fully present in the moment, is a powerful tool in achieving balance. Incorporating mindfulness techniques into daily routines, such as meditation or mindful breathing, fosters a heightened awareness that can alleviate stress and enhance overall well-being.

Empowering Others:

Empowering colleagues and collaborators contributes to a positive work environment. By fostering a culture of support and collaboration, working women can create a more inclusive and empathetic professional landscape that values well-being alongside achievement.

Embracing Imperfection:

Accepting that perfection is an unattainable standard is liberating. Embracing imperfection allows for greater self-compassion, reducing the self-imposed pressure to excel in every facet of life.

Conclusion

The pursuit of a balanced life for working women is not a destination but a continual journey. It requires adaptability, resilience, and a commitment to ongoing self-discovery. By acknowledging the interconnectedness of work and well-being and implementing intentional strategies, women can navigate the challenges of the modern workplace while nurturing their physical, mental, and emotional health. The balancing act is not a compromise but a harmonious integration of professional success and personal fulfillment, creating a sustainable and fulfilling life.

Chapter 2

Nourishing Your Body and Mind

Amidst the Hustle

Introduction:

In the bustling world of deadlines, meetings, and constant connectivity, the quest for nourishing both body and mind can often seem like an elusive goal. Yet, it is precisely amidst the hustle of daily life that the importance of self-care becomes paramount. Nourishing your body and mind is not a luxury; it's a fundamental investment in your well-being that pays dividends in both personal and professional realms.

The Neglected Foundations: Nutrition and Hydration

Amidst the chaos of hectic schedules, proper nutrition and hydration often take a backseat. Fast food, skipped meals, and inadequate water intake become commonplace as individuals prioritize work over their own sustenance. However, neglecting these foundational elements can have far-reaching consequences on both physical and mental health.

Fueling Your Body:

Adequate nutrition is the fuel that powers your body through the demands of a busy day. Incorporating a balanced diet rich in whole foods provides essential nutrients that support energy levels, cognitive function, and overall vitality. Simple changes, such as packing nutritious snacks or preparing wholesome meals in advance, can significantly enhance your ability to navigate the hustle without compromising your health.

Hydration as a Cornerstone:

Water is not only the elixir of life but also a cornerstone of well-being. Dehydration can lead to fatigue, impaired concentration, and a decline in physical performance. Cultivating the habit of regular hydration, perhaps by keeping a water bottle at your desk or setting reminders, is a small yet powerful step toward nourishing your body amidst the demands of a busy lifestyle.

Mindful Eating in a Fast-Paced World

The concept of mindful eating is a beacon of sanity in a world characterized by hurried meals and mindless consumption. It involves savoring each bite, paying attention to the sensory experience of eating, and cultivating a deeper connection with the food on your plate.

Breaking Free from Multitasking:

In a culture that glorifies multitasking, mealtimes often become an extension of work or other activities. Mindful eating encourages breaking free from this pattern. Instead of hastily consuming meals while glued to a screen or engrossed in work, take a few minutes to savor each bite without distractions. This simple shift in approach can enhance your appreciation for food and contribute to a more mindful relationship with nourishment.

Understanding Hunger and Fullness:

Mindful eating involves tuning in to your body's signals of hunger and fullness. Rather than eating on autopilot or following external cues, listen to your body's needs. This awareness can help prevent overeating and foster a healthier relationship with food.

Choosing Quality Over Quantity:

The hustle often tempts us to opt for convenience over quality when it comes to food choices. However, prioritizing nutrient-dense, whole foods over processed alternatives is a conscious decision that can positively impact your overall health. Consider incorporating fruits, vegetables, whole grains, and lean proteins into your meals, even in the midst of a busy schedule.

Cultivating Mental Nourishment: Strategies for Mind Wellness

While nourishing the body is essential, fostering mental well-being is equally crucial amidst the hustle. The relentless pace of modern life, coupled with constant demands, can take a toll on mental health. Cultivating practices that nurture your mind is an investment in resilience, focus, and emotional balance.

Moments of Mindfulness:

Incorporating mindfulness practices into your daily routine can be transformative. Whether through meditation, deep breathing exercises, or simply taking moments of quiet reflection, mindfulness allows you to anchor yourself in the present moment. Amidst the hustle, these moments become invaluable, providing a respite from the chaos and promoting mental clarity.

Strategic Breaks for Mental Renewal:

The misconception that constant work leads to increased productivity is debunked by the science of productivity. Strategic breaks, even if brief, can enhance cognitive function and creativity. Schedule short breaks during the day to step away from your work, stretch, or engage in a quick mindfulness exercise. These breaks serve as mental reset buttons, allowing you to return to your tasks with renewed focus and energy.

Digital Detox for Mental Clarity:

The omnipresence of digital devices can contribute to mental fatigue. A digital detox, even if temporary, can be rejuvenating. Designate specific times to disconnect from screens, especially before bedtime, to promote better sleep quality and reduce mental clutter. This intentional break from constant connectivity fosters a sense of mental spaciousness.

Cultivating a Growth Mindset:

The mindset with which you approach challenges significantly influences your well-being. Embracing a growth mindset, which sees challenges as opportunities for learning and development, can enhance resilience amidst the hustle. Rather than viewing obstacles as insurmountable, see them as stepping stones to personal and professional growth.

Connecting with Passions:

Amidst work obligations, it's crucial to carve out time for activities that bring joy and fulfillment. Whether it's a hobby, creative pursuit, or simply spending time in nature, connecting with your passions is a form of mental nourishment. These activities serve as an antidote to stress and contribute to a more balanced and contented mind.

Physical Activity: A Pillar of Well-being

In the midst of a demanding schedule, the inclination to prioritize physical activity can wane. However, regular exercise is not only essential for physical health but is also a potent tool for managing stress, enhancing mood, and promoting overall well-being.

Incorporating Movement into Daily Life:

The misconception that exercise requires lengthy gym sessions contributes to its neglect. Incorporating movement into your daily routine, such as taking the stairs, going for short walks, or engaging in quick home workouts, is a practical way to prioritize physical activity. These micro-movements accumulate and contribute to improved fitness over time.

Choosing Activities, You Enjoy:

The hustle becomes more manageable when physical activity aligns with your interests. Whether it's dancing, cycling, yoga, or team sports, choosing activities you enjoy transforms exercise from a chore into a source of pleasure. This not only enhances consistency but also adds an element of joy to your routine.

Prioritizing Consistency Over Intensity:

In the midst of a busy schedule, the consistency of physical activity outweighs its intensity. Short, regular workouts are more sustainable and yield long-term benefits. Establishing a realistic exercise routine that accommodates your lifestyle ensures that physical activity remains a non-negotiable aspect of your well-being.

Strategies for Implementation: Turning Intentions into Action

Nourishing your body and mind requires intentional actions that align with your goals and priorities. Implementing these strategies amidst the hustle of daily life may seem challenging, but with a systematic approach, it becomes not only feasible but transformative.

Creating a Well-being Plan:

Develop a well-being plan that outlines your goals for physical and mental health. Clearly define actionable steps, such as specific meal choices, exercise routines, and mindfulness practices. Having a written plan provides a roadmap for implementation and serves as a tangible reminder of your commitment to well-being.

Scheduling Self-Care Time:

Treat self-care as a non-negotiable appointment in your calendar. Schedule time for meals, breaks, exercise, and mindfulness just as you would schedule work-related tasks. This intentional approach ensures that self-care becomes a prioritized aspect of your daily routine.

Building a Support System:

Share your well-being goals with friends, family, or colleagues who can offer support and accountability. Having a support system creates a sense of collective commitment to well-being, making it more likely that you'll stay on track.

Adapting to Change:

Recognize that the demands of the hustle may vary from day to day. Be flexible in adapting your well-being practices to suit different circumstances. Whether it's adjusting your exercise routine or choosing quick and nutritious meal options, adaptability is key to sustainable well-being.

Celebrating Small Wins:

Acknowledge and celebrate the small victories along the way. Whether it's consistently incorporating mindfulness into your day or making healthier food choices, recognizing these achievements reinforces positive habits and motivates continued efforts.

Conclusion: Thriving Amidst the Hustle

In the relentless pace of modern life, the art of nourishing your body and mind amidst the hustle is a transformative practice that goes beyond mere survival. It is a commitment to thriving in the face of challenges, cultivating resilience, and prioritizing well-being as a fundamental aspect of a fulfilling life.

By recognizing the interconnectedness of physical and mental health, embracing mindful practices, and prioritizing self-care in practical ways, you not only enhance your ability to navigate the demands of a busy lifestyle but also contribute to sustained success and happiness. The journey of nourishment amidst the hustle is a personal and empowering one, reminding you that amidst the chaos, you have the power to prioritize your well-being and thrive in every aspect of life.

Chapter 3

Crafting a Sustainable Work-Life Harmony

Introduction:

In the ever-evolving landscape of the professional world, the pursuit of a harmonious balance between work and life has become an essential aspiration. Rather than a mere juggling act, the concept of work-life harmony embodies the intentional crafting of an integrated and sustainable lifestyle that nurtures both professional and personal fulfillment. This approach acknowledges that the traditional notion of a strict work-life balance may not be achievable or desirable in today's dynamic and interconnected world.

Redefining Work-Life Harmony
Shift from Balance to Harmony:

The term "balance" often implies an equal distribution of weight or effort, suggesting that work and life are opposing forces that need to be counteracted. Work-life harmony, on the other hand, acknowledges the dynamic interplay between the two. It recognizes that achieving perfect equilibrium may be unrealistic and, instead, focuses on integrating the various facets of life into a cohesive and sustainable whole.

The Myth of Perfect Balance:

Striving for a perfect balance can lead to frustration and stress. The demands of work and personal life are fluid and constantly changing, making it challenging to maintain a static equilibrium. Embracing the idea of harmony allows for flexibility and adaptation to the ebb and flow of life's demands.

Elements of Sustainable Work-Life Harmony Clarifying Priorities:

Crafting a sustainable work-life harmony begins with a clear understanding of your values and priorities. Identify the aspects of both work and personal life that are most meaningful to you. This clarity serves as a guiding framework for decision-making and resource allocation.

Defining Success on Your Terms:

Societal definitions of success often revolve around external achievements and recognition. However, crafting work-life harmony involves defining success on your own terms. What brings you a sense of accomplishment and fulfillment may differ from conventional benchmarks. Align your goals with your personal values rather than external expectations.

Establishing Boundaries:

Boundaries are the cornerstone of a sustainable work-life harmony. Clearly delineate the limits between work and personal time, both physically and mentally. This may involve setting specific working hours, designating work-free zones in your home, and communicating your boundaries to colleagues and family members.

Embracing Flexibility:

The rigidity of traditional work structures is often antithetical to achieving harmony. Embracing flexibility in work arrangements, such as remote work options or flexible hours, can empower individuals to tailor their work environments to suit their personal needs. This adaptability is instrumental in responding to the changing demands of both work and life.

Mindful Time Management:

Time management is a critical skill in crafting work-life harmony. However, it's not just about managing time; it's about managing energy and attention. Prioritize tasks based on their significance and allocate focused time for both work and personal pursuits. Implementing techniques like the Pomodoro method or time blocking can enhance productivity while maintaining a sense of balance.

Investing in Self-Care:

Sustainable work-life harmony necessitates a commitment to self-care. Prioritizing physical health, mental well-being, and emotional resilience is not a luxury but a foundational element of overall harmony. This may include regular exercise, sufficient sleep, and activities that bring joy and relaxation.

Cultivating Interpersonal Relationships:

Meaningful connections with family, friends, and colleagues contribute to a sense of fulfillment. Investing time in nurturing interpersonal relationships strengthens your support system and provides a valuable counterbalance to the demands of work. Quality relationships enhance both personal and professional well-being.

Continuous Learning and Growth:

Work-life harmony involves an ongoing process of learning and personal development. Cultivating a growth mindset, staying curious, and acquiring new skills contribute to a sense of progress and fulfillment. This commitment to growth extends beyond the professional realm, encompassing personal interests and passions.

Navigating Challenges:

Overcoming Guilt and Expectations:

Guilt often accompanies the pursuit of work-life harmony, especially when societal expectations or workplace cultures prioritize constant availability. Overcoming this guilt requires a shift in mindset. Recognize that prioritizing your well-being enhances your effectiveness both at work and in personal life.

Communication and Advocacy:

Effectively communicating your needs and boundaries is essential in navigating challenges. Whether negotiating flexible work arrangements with your employer or communicating personal commitments to colleagues, proactive communication fosters understanding and support.

Managing Burnout:

Burnout is a significant risk in high-pressure environments. Recognizing the signs of burnout, such as chronic fatigue and diminished enthusiasm, is crucial. Implementing strategies like regular breaks, delegation of tasks, and seeking support when needed can prevent and mitigate burnout.

Technology and Disconnecting:

The pervasive nature of technology can blur the lines between work and personal life. Establishing designated times to disconnect from devices and work-related communication helps create a clear distinction between work and leisure. This intentional break is vital for mental rejuvenation.

Success Stories and Inspirations:
Company Culture that Values Harmony:

Some forward-thinking companies recognize the importance of work-life harmony and have implemented policies that support their employees' well-being. Whether through flexible work hours, remote work options, or wellness programs, these companies prioritize a holistic approach to employee satisfaction.

Individuals Who Have Mastered Harmony:

Exploring the stories of individuals who have successfully crafted work-life harmony can provide valuable insights and inspiration. These individuals often share common themes of prioritizing their values, setting boundaries, and embracing flexibility. Learning from their experiences can offer practical strategies for achieving harmony in your own life.

Conclusion:

Crafting a sustainable work-life harmony is not a one-time achievement but a continual process of self-discovery and adaptation. It requires a mindful and intentional approach to aligning your professional and personal pursuits with your values and priorities. By redefining success, establishing boundaries, embracing flexibility, and prioritizing self-care, individuals can navigate the complexities of the modern world while fostering a sense of fulfillment and balance.

In this ongoing journey, the key lies in recognizing that work and life are not competing forces but complementary elements of a holistic and meaningful existence. As individuals continue to craft their unique paths to work-life harmony, they contribute not only to their personal well-being but also to a cultural shift that values fulfillment, resilience, and a sustainable approach to success.

Chapter 4

The Power of Mindfulness: Stress Management Techniques

Introduction:

In the fast-paced and demanding landscape of today's world, stress has become a ubiquitous companion for many. As the pressures of work, personal responsibilities, and societal expectations intensify, the need for effective stress management techniques becomes increasingly imperative. At the forefront of these techniques lies mindfulness – a practice that not only addresses the symptoms of stress but also cultivates a profound shift in the way individuals relate to and perceive the challenges they face.

Understanding Mindfulness:
A Present-Moment Focus:

At its core, mindfulness is the practice of being fully present in the moment, without judgment. It involves directing one's attention to the current experience, whether it be sensations, thoughts, or emotions, with a non-reactive and accepting mindset. By anchoring awareness in the present, individuals can break free from the cycle of stress-inducing thoughts about the past or future.

Mindfulness Meditation:

A cornerstone of mindfulness is meditation, which involves dedicating a specific time to engage in focused awareness. This can take various forms, such as guided meditation, body scan, or breath awareness. Regular mindfulness meditation sessions have been shown to have a transformative impact on stress levels, promoting a sense of calm and resilience.

Bringing Mindfulness into Daily Life:

Mindfulness extends beyond formal meditation sessions. Integrating mindfulness into daily activities – from eating to walking – can be equally powerful. This involves approaching routine tasks with full attention and intention, fostering a heightened awareness of the present moment.

The Science Behind Mindfulness and Stress Reduction:

Impact on the Brain:

Scientific research has demonstrated that mindfulness practices can lead to structural changes in the brain, particularly in areas associated with emotional regulation and stress response. The amygdala, a key player in the brain's stress system, shows reduced activity with regular mindfulness practice, contributing to a diminished perception of stress.

Cortisol Regulation:

Mindfulness has been linked to improved regulation of cortisol, the primary stress hormone. Chronic stress often results in elevated cortisol levels, which can have detrimental effects on physical and mental health. Mindfulness practices have been shown to modulate cortisol secretion, promoting a more balanced and adaptive stress response.

Enhanced Emotional Regulation:

Mindfulness equips individuals with the tools to observe their emotions without being overwhelmed by them. This enhanced emotional awareness and regulation contribute to a more measured response to stressors, reducing the intensity and duration of stress-related reactions.

Mindfulness-Based Stress Reduction (MBSR):

Structured Programs for Stress Reduction:

Developed by Dr. Jon Kabat-Zinn, Mindfulness-Based Stress Reduction (MBSR) is a structured program that combines mindfulness meditation and yoga to alleviate stress. MBSR has been widely adopted in various settings, from healthcare institutions to corporate wellness programs, as a comprehensive approach to stress management.

Components of MBSR:

MBSR typically involves a series of sessions that guide participants through mindfulness meditation, gentle yoga, and discussions on stress, resilience, and mindful living. The program emphasizes cultivating a non-judgmental awareness of thoughts and feelings, fostering a compassionate attitude toward oneself and others.

Mindfulness in the Workplace:

Enhancing Focus and Productivity:

In a work environment characterized by constant demands and distractions, mindfulness has emerged as a valuable tool for enhancing focus and productivity. Short mindfulness exercises, such as brief meditation sessions or mindful breathing, can be incorporated into the workday to help individuals center themselves and improve concentration.

Stress Reduction in Corporate Settings:

Forward-thinking companies are recognizing the importance of employee well-being and incorporating mindfulness initiatives into their corporate cultures. From offering mindfulness workshops to providing designated meditation spaces, these initiatives aim to reduce workplace stress and foster a more positive and resilient workforce.

Practical Mindfulness Techniques for Stress Management:

Mindful Breathing:

One of the simplest yet most powerful mindfulness techniques is mindful breathing. Taking a few minutes to focus on the breath – inhaling and exhaling consciously – can have an immediate calming effect. This technique can be practiced anywhere, making it a versatile tool for on-the-spot stress management.

Body Scan Meditation:

Body scan meditation involves systematically directing attention to different parts of the body, noticing sensations without judgment. This practice promotes a heightened awareness of bodily tension and provides an opportunity for relaxation.

Regular body scan sessions can contribute to overall stress reduction.

Mindful Walking:

Incorporating mindfulness into physical activity, such as walking, adds a dynamic dimension to the practice. Paying attention to each step, the sensations of movement, and the surrounding environment can transform a routine activity into a mindfulness exercise. This technique is particularly useful for those who find sitting meditation challenging.

Mindful Eating:

In a culture where meals are often rushed or consumed in front of screens, mindful eating encourages a more intentional and present approach to nourishment. Paying attention to the colors, textures, and flavors of food, as well as the act of chewing, enhances the dining experience and promotes a sense of satisfaction.

Mindful Technology Use:

The pervasive use of digital devices can contribute to stress and mental clutter. Mindful technology use involves setting intentional boundaries for device use, taking breaks from screens, and being fully present during interactions. This practice supports a healthier relationship with technology and reduces the cognitive load associated with constant connectivity.

Challenges and Misconceptions:

Patience and Consistency:

One of the challenges individuals may face in adopting mindfulness practices is the need for patience and consistency. The benefits of mindfulness often unfold gradually, requiring regular practice over time. Establishing a consistent routine, even if it involves short sessions, is key to experiencing the full impact of mindfulness on stress management.

Misconceptions about Mindfulness:

Mindfulness is sometimes misunderstood as a passive state of relaxation or as a technique that requires emptying the mind of thoughts. In reality, mindfulness involves an active and non-judgmental awareness of the present moment, which includes acknowledging and observing thoughts without becoming entangled in them.

Cultivating a Mindful Lifestyle:

Mindful Communication:

Mindfulness extends to interpersonal interactions, shaping the way individuals communicate. Mindful communication involves listening with full attention, speaking with intention, and fostering empathy. This approach contributes to healthier relationships and reduces the stress associated with miscommunication.

Gratitude Practices:

Gratitude is intertwined with mindfulness, as both involve cultivating a positive and appreciative outlook on life. Engaging in gratitude practices, such as keeping a gratitude journal or expressing appreciation for small moments, contributes to a sense of well-being and resilience in the face of stress.

Mindfulness in Difficult Moments:

The true test of mindfulness occurs in challenging situations. The ability to bring mindfulness into moments of difficulty – whether it's a stressful meeting, a conflict, or an unexpected setback – empowers individuals to respond with greater clarity and composure.

Conclusion: Empowerment through Mindfulness

In the face of the stressors that characterize contemporary life, the power of mindfulness lies in its capacity to empower individuals to respond to challenges with greater resilience, awareness, and equanimity. As a holistic approach to stress management, mindfulness not only addresses the symptoms but also instills a transformative shift in the way individuals perceive and engage with their experiences.

By integrating mindfulness into daily life, both through formal practices and moment-to-moment awareness, individuals can cultivate a sustainable foundation for stress management. As the science of mindfulness continues to unfold and its applications expand, the recognition of its potential to enhance well-being and foster a balanced, harmonious life becomes increasingly evident. Ultimately, the power of mindfulness lies in its invitation to reclaim the present moment, find stillness amidst chaos, and rediscover a sense of agency in the face of life's inevitable challenges.

Chapter 5

Fitness on the Fly: Quick Workouts for Busy Schedules

In the hustle and bustle of modern life, finding time for a comprehensive workout routine can be a formidable challenge. Busy schedules, work commitments, and family responsibilities often leave little room for extended gym sessions or lengthy exercise regimens. However, the importance of regular physical activity for overall health and well-being cannot be overstated. The solution lies in embracing the concept of "Fitness on the Fly" – a strategy that involves incorporating quick and effective workouts into the busiest of schedules.

The Significance of Physical Activity:

Beyond Aesthetics:

While achieving fitness goals and maintaining a desirable physique are common motivators for exercise, the benefits of physical activity extend far beyond aesthetics. Regular exercise is linked to improved cardiovascular health, enhanced mood, better sleep, and increased energy levels. These holistic advantages underscore the importance of finding practical ways to integrate fitness into daily life.

Stress Reduction:

Physical activity is a potent stress reliever. In the midst of hectic schedules and constant demands, a brief workout can serve as a powerful antidote to stress. Exercise triggers the release of endorphins, the body's natural mood elevators, promoting a sense of well-being and mental clarity.

Boosting Productivity:

Contrary to the belief that exercise consumes precious time, incorporating quick workouts can actually boost productivity. The enhanced focus and increased energy levels that result from physical activity can positively impact work performance, making the time invested in exercise a valuable investment in overall efficiency.

The Fitness on the Fly Approach:

Short Bursts of Activity:

Fitness on the Fly revolves around the idea of short, intense bursts of activity that can be seamlessly integrated into a busy day. These workouts are designed to maximize efficiency, focusing on compound movements and high-intensity intervals to deliver a comprehensive workout in a condensed timeframe.

Minimal Equipment:

The beauty of Fitness on the Fly lies in its minimalistic approach to equipment. Many of these workouts can be performed using bodyweight exercises, requiring little to no additional equipment. This eliminates the need for a dedicated gym space and allows individuals to exercise in the comfort of their homes or even at the workplace.

Adaptability to Any Setting:

Whether you're traveling, working late, or facing a time crunch, Fitness on the Fly is adaptable to any setting. These workouts can be customized to fit into various environments, making it a versatile approach that doesn't require a fixed location or specialized equipment.

Quick Workouts for Busy Schedules:

High-Intensity Interval Training (HIIT):

HIIT is a cornerstone of Fitness on the Fly, combining short bursts of intense exercise with brief periods of rest or lower-intensity activity. A 15 to 20-minute HIIT session can effectively elevate heart rate, burn calories, and improve cardiovascular fitness. Sample exercises include jumping jacks, burpees, mountain climbers, and high knees.

Tabata Training:

Tabata is a specific form of HIIT that involves 20 seconds of all-out effort followed by 10 seconds of rest, repeated for four minutes. This protocol can be applied to exercises like squats, push-ups, or sprints. Tabata is known for its efficiency, delivering a substantial workout in a minimal amount of time.

Bodyweight Circuits:

Bodyweight circuits involve performing a series of exercises consecutively with minimal rest between each. These circuits can target different muscle groups and provide a full-body workout. A sample circuit may include squats, lunges, push-ups, planks, and jumping jacks. Completing two to three rounds of such a circuit can be a time-efficient yet effective workout.

Quick Cardio Blasts:

When time is of the essence, short cardio bursts can be incredibly effective. This can include a quick session of jump rope, a series of sprints, or even stair climbing. These activities elevate heart rate rapidly, providing cardiovascular benefits in a condensed timeframe.

Power Yoga or Pilates:

Yoga and Pilates are excellent options for Fitness on the Fly, as they combine strength, flexibility, and mindfulness. Short power yoga or Pilates sessions can be tailored to focus on specific areas, providing a quick yet holistic workout.

Resistance Band Exercises:

Portable and versatile, resistance bands offer an effective way to add resistance to bodyweight exercises. Squats, lunges, rows, and bicep curls can all be enhanced with the use of resistance bands. These exercises target muscle groups efficiently and can be incorporated into a time-efficient workout routine.

Quick Core Workouts:

Core strength is fundamental to overall fitness. Quick core workouts, featuring exercises like planks, Russian twists, leg raises, and bicycle crunches, can be performed in a matter of minutes yet provide substantial benefits for abdominal strength and stability.

Strategies for Incorporating Fitness on the Fly:

Schedule It:

Treat your workout as an essential appointment by scheduling it into your daily calendar. Whether it's a lunchtime routine, a quick session before work, or a brief workout during a break, having a designated time increases the likelihood of consistency.

Make It a Habit:

Consistency is key to seeing results. Establishing a habit of incorporating Fitness on the Fly into your routine makes it more likely that exercise becomes an automatic part of your day. Start with small, manageable goals and gradually increase intensity and duration.

Maximize Breaks:

Use breaks during the workday as opportunities for quick physical activity. Whether it's a brisk walk, a set of squats, or a brief stretch routine, these micro-workouts can contribute to overall fitness without disrupting the flow of your day.

Utilize Technology:

Fitness apps and online resources offer a plethora of quick workout routines. From guided HIIT sessions to yoga flows, leveraging technology can provide structure and variety to your Fitness on the Fly approach.

Combine Activities:

Look for opportunities to combine exercise with other activities. For example, take the stairs instead of the elevator, perform bodyweight exercises while waiting for appointments, or incorporate quick stretches into your daily routine. This multi-tasking approach maximizes time efficiency.

Overcoming Common Challenges:

Overcoming Perfectionism:

The notion that a workout must be lengthy or intense can hinder individuals from embracing shorter, more frequent sessions. Overcoming perfectionism involves recognizing the value of consistency and acknowledging that even brief workouts contribute to overall well-being.

Creating a Supportive Environment:

Surround yourself with a supportive environment that encourages physical activity. This could involve enlisting a workout buddy, joining fitness groups, or finding online communities that share your commitment to Fitness on the Fly.

Prioritizing Self-Care:

Recognize that exercise is a form of self-care and not a luxury. Prioritizing your well-being, even in the midst of a busy schedule, is an investment in your physical and mental health. The benefits of exercise extend beyond the immediate timeframe, contributing to sustained energy and resilience.

Conclusion:

Fitness on the Fly offers a pragmatic and sustainable approach to incorporating physical activity into the busiest of lifestyles. By redefining the traditional notion of lengthy workouts and embracing the efficiency of short, targeted sessions, individuals can prioritize their health without compromising on productivity.

The key lies in making fitness a seamless part of daily life, recognizing that even brief moments of movement contribute to overall well-being. As the world continues to move at an accelerated pace, the value of Fitness on the Fly becomes increasingly evident — not just as a time-saving strategy but as a holistic approach to health that aligns with the demands of contemporary living. So, whether it's a quick HIIT session in the morning, a brief yoga flow during lunch, or a short cardio burst in the evening, the power of Fitness on the Fly lies in its accessibility, efficiency, and transformative impact on physical and mental vitality.

Chapter 6

Mindful Eating Strategies for Busy Professionals: Nourishing Your Body and Mind in the Midst of Chaos

Introduction:

In the fast-paced world of today's professionals, maintaining a healthy and balanced lifestyle often takes a back seat to the demands of work. One aspect that is frequently neglected is mindful eating, which involves being fully present and aware during meals. For busy professionals, incorporating mindful eating strategies into their routine can be transformative, leading to improved overall well-being. This article explores the importance of mindful eating, its benefits, and provides practical strategies for busy professionals to cultivate this practice in their daily lives.

The Importance of Mindful Eating:

Mindful eating is not just a trendy concept; it's a holistic approach to nourishing both the body and mind. In a society dominated by multitasking and constant connectivity, many individuals find themselves consuming meals in a rushed and distracted manner. This can contribute to overeating, poor digestion, and a general disconnect from the sensory experience of eating.

By contrast, mindful eating encourages individuals to engage their senses, pay attention to the textures and flavors of their food, and recognize the signals of hunger and fullness. This heightened awareness fosters a healthier relationship with food and promotes a sense of satisfaction that goes beyond mere calorie intake.

Benefits of Mindful Eating for Busy Professionals:

Improved Digestion:

Mindful eating encourages chewing food thoroughly, aiding in better digestion and nutrient absorption.

Being present during meals helps the body enter a relaxed state, promoting optimal digestive function.

Weight Management:

Mindful eating can prevent overeating by enhancing awareness of hunger and fullness cues.

Individuals are more likely to make healthier food choices when they are attuned to their body's needs.

Stress Reduction:

Taking the time to enjoy meals without distractions can be a powerful stress management tool.

Mindful eating shifts the focus from external stressors to the present moment, promoting a sense of calm.

Increased Energy Levels:

Proper digestion and nutrient absorption from mindful eating contribute to sustained energy levels throughout the day.

Choosing nutrient-dense foods in a mindful manner provides the body with the fuel it needs.

Enhanced Focus and Productivity:

Mindful eating breaks allow professionals to reset and recharge, leading to improved focus and productivity.

The practice cultivates a mindful mindset that can be applied to other aspects of work and life.

Practical Mindful Eating Strategies for Busy Professionals:

Set aside dedicated meal times:

Block out specific times for meals in your schedule and treat them as non-negotiable appointments.

Avoid working through lunch or eating at your desk; instead, create a designated space for mindful eating.

Minimize distractions:

Turn off electronic devices, including phones and computers, during meals.

Create a serene environment by eating in a quiet space, free from the hustle and bustle of work.

Practice gratitude before meals:

Take a moment to express gratitude for the food in front of you, acknowledging the effort and resources that went into its creation.

This practice sets a positive tone for the meal and encourages mindful awareness.

Chew slowly and savor each bite:

Pay attention to the texture, taste, and aroma of your food.

Chew each bite thoroughly, allowing the digestive process to begin in the mouth.

Listen to your body's signals:

Pause during the meal to assess your hunger and fullness levels.

Avoid eating beyond the point of fullness, and trust your body's cues.

Choose nutrient-dense foods:

Opt for whole, unprocessed foods that nourish your body and provide sustained energy.

Be mindful of portion sizes and make conscious choices about the quality of the food you consume.

Plan and prepare meals in advance:

Allocate time for meal planning and preparation to ensure you have nourishing options readily available.

Having healthy meals on hand reduces the temptation to grab convenience foods that may not align with mindful eating.

Practice mindful breathing:

Take a few deep breaths before starting your meal to center yourself and transition from work mode to a more mindful state.

Incorporate mindful breathing between bites to stay present and focused.

Create mindful eating rituals:

Establish rituals, such as setting a beautifully arranged table or using special utensils, to enhance the sensory experience of eating.

Rituals signal the transition from work to nourishment and can make meals more enjoyable.

Stay flexible and be forgiving:

Understand that there will be days when the demands of work may disrupt your ideal eating routine.

Be forgiving of yourself and aim to return to mindful eating when circumstances allow.

Conclusion:

In the whirlwind of professional responsibilities, it's easy to neglect the simple yet profound act of eating. Mindful eating offers a pathway for busy professionals to reconnect with their bodies, prioritize their well-being, and foster a healthier relationship with food. By incorporating these mindful eating strategies into their daily lives, professionals can not only enhance their physical health but also improve their mental clarity, productivity, and overall quality of life. In the midst of chaos, mindful eating becomes a grounding practice that nourishes both the body and mind, creating a harmonious balance in the demanding world of busy professionals.

Chapter 7

Building Resilience: A Comprehensive Guide to Coping with Workplace Challenges

Introduction:

In the dynamic and often stressful landscape of the modern workplace, building resilience has become a crucial skill for professionals to navigate and thrive amidst challenges. Resilience is the ability to bounce back from setbacks, adapt to change, and maintain a positive outlook in the face of adversity. This article explores the significance of resilience in the workplace, identifies common challenges professionals encounter, and provides a comprehensive guide on building and enhancing resilience to cope effectively with these challenges.

The Importance of Resilience in the Workplace:

Adaptability to Change:

Resilience allows individuals to embrace change and view it as an opportunity for growth rather than a threat.

In rapidly evolving work environments, adaptability is a key factor in long-term success.

Stress Management:

Resilient individuals are better equipped to manage stress, preventing it from escalating into chronic issues such as burnout.

The ability to cope with stress positively impacts mental and physical well-being.

Enhanced Problem-Solving:

Resilience fosters a problem-solving mindset, enabling professionals to approach challenges with creativity and resourcefulness.

This skill is essential for overcoming obstacles and finding innovative solutions.

Positive Work Relationships:

Resilient individuals maintain positive interpersonal relationships, even in the face of disagreements or conflicts.

Building and sustaining healthy connections with colleagues contributes to a supportive work environment.

Increased Productivity:

The ability to bounce back from setbacks reduces the time spent dwelling on challenges, allowing professionals to remain focused and productive.

Resilient individuals are more likely to persevere through difficulties, leading to increased task completion.

Common Workplace Challenges:

High Workload and Tight Deadlines:

Professionals often face the pressure of managing heavy workloads and meeting tight deadlines.

The stress associated with these demands can impact both mental and physical health.

Interpersonal Conflicts:

Workplace relationships may be strained due to differences in communication styles, conflicting priorities, or misunderstandings.

Navigating interpersonal conflicts requires resilience to maintain a positive work environment.

Job Insecurity:

Economic uncertainties, industry changes, or company restructuring can lead to job insecurity.

Fear of job loss can significantly impact job performance and overall well-being.

Lack of Recognition:

Professionals may feel demotivated when their efforts go unnoticed or unappreciated.

A lack of recognition can erode morale and hinder job satisfaction.

Organizational Changes:

Mergers, acquisitions, or shifts in leadership can create uncertainty and disrupt established workflows.

Resilience is crucial for adapting to organizational changes and maintaining stability.

Work-Life Imbalance:

Juggling professional responsibilities with personal commitments can lead to work-life imbalance.

Striking a harmonious balance requires resilience to manage competing priorities.

Building and Enhancing Resilience:

Cultivate a Growth Mindset:

Embrace challenges as opportunities for learning and growth.

View setbacks as temporary and focus on the lessons they provide.

Develop Strong Interpersonal Skills:

Build effective communication and conflict resolution skills to navigate workplace relationships.

Foster a supportive network of colleagues who can provide guidance and encouragement.

Set Realistic Goals:

Break down larger goals into smaller, manageable tasks.

Celebrate small victories, reinforcing a sense of accomplishment and progress.

Prioritize Self-Care:

Establish a routine that includes regular breaks, sufficient sleep, and exercise.

Attend to both physical and mental well-being to enhance overall resilience.

Seek Professional Development:

Continuously invest in learning and acquiring new skills.

Staying relevant in your field builds confidence and adaptability.

Maintain a Positive Mindset:

Focus on positive aspects of your work and life.

Practice gratitude to cultivate a positive outlook, even in challenging situations.

Build a Support System:

Connect with colleagues, mentors, or support groups.

Sharing experiences and seeking advice can provide valuable perspectives.

Develop Problem-Solving Skills:

Approach challenges methodically, breaking them down into manageable components.

Seek input from colleagues and consider alternative solutions.

Foster Flexibility:

Embrace change and approach it with an open mind.

Develop the ability to adapt to new circumstances and adjust plans accordingly.

Set Boundaries:

Clearly define professional and personal boundaries.

Communicate expectations regarding workload and commitments to maintain a healthy work-life balance.

Conclusion:

In the ever-evolving landscape of the workplace, building resilience is not just a desirable skill but a necessity for professional success and well-being. By understanding the importance of resilience, recognizing common workplace challenges, and implementing practical strategies for building and enhancing resilience, professionals can navigate their careers with greater confidence and effectiveness. Resilience empowers individuals to transform adversity into opportunities, fostering personal and professional growth. As professionals embrace the journey of building resilience, they not only enhance their own capacity to thrive but also contribute to creating resilient and adaptive workplaces.

Chapter 8

Sleep Smart: The Foundation of a Productive Day

Introduction:

In the bustling world of modern life, where productivity is often a badge of honor, the importance of quality sleep cannot be overstated. Sleep is not merely a luxury; it is a fundamental pillar of physical and mental well-being. This article delves into the critical role of sleep in overall health, explores the impact of sleep on productivity, and provides practical strategies for adopting smart sleep habits to lay the foundation for a more productive day.

Understanding the Importance of Quality Sleep:

Physical Restoration:

During sleep, the body undergoes crucial processes of repair and restoration.

Muscles are repaired, tissues are regenerated, and the immune system is strengthened, contributing to overall physical health.

Cognitive Function:

Sleep plays a vital role in cognitive functions such as memory consolidation, problem-solving, and learning.

Lack of sleep can impair concentration, decision-making, and the ability to process information effectively.

Emotional Well-being:

Adequate sleep is linked to emotional resilience and stability.

Sleep deficiency is associated with an increased risk of mood disorders, anxiety, and heightened emotional reactivity.

Metabolic Balance:

Quality sleep is crucial for maintaining a healthy metabolism and weight.

Sleep deprivation can disrupt hormonal balance, leading to increased cravings for unhealthy foods and a higher risk of obesity.

Cardiovascular Health:

Chronic sleep deprivation is linked to an elevated risk of cardiovascular diseases.

Adequate sleep supports heart health by regulating blood pressure and reducing inflammation.

The Impact of Sleep on Productivity:

Enhanced Cognitive Performance:

Quality sleep is directly linked to improved cognitive functions, including memory retention, problem-solving, and creativity.

Professionals who prioritize sleep often experience heightened focus and mental clarity.

Increased Efficiency:

Adequate rest contributes to increased efficiency and productivity during working hours.

Well-rested individuals can accomplish tasks more quickly and accurately compared to those who are sleep-deprived.

Better Decision-Making:

Sleep plays a crucial role in executive functions, enabling individuals to make sound decisions and solve complex problems.

Sleep-deprived individuals are more prone to impulsivity and poor judgment.

Effective Stress Management:

Quality sleep is a natural stress buster, helping individuals cope with daily challenges more effectively.

Sleep-deprived individuals often experience heightened stress levels and reduced resilience.

Improved Interpersonal Skills:

Lack of sleep can impact communication skills and the ability to collaborate effectively.

Well-rested individuals are better equipped to navigate workplace relationships and communicate with clarity.

Practical Strategies for Smart Sleep:

Establish a Consistent Sleep Schedule:

Go to bed and wake up at the same time every day, even on weekends.

Consistency reinforces the body's natural circadian rhythm, promoting better sleep quality.

Create a Relaxing Bedtime Routine:

Develop a calming pre-sleep routine to signal to your body that it's time to wind down.

Activities such as reading, gentle stretching, or listening to soothing music can help prepare the mind for rest.

Optimize Your Sleep Environment:

Ensure your bedroom is conducive to sleep by keeping it cool, dark, and quiet.

Invest in a comfortable mattress and pillows to promote a restful night's sleep.

Limit Exposure to Screens Before Bed:

Reduce exposure to screens (phones, tablets, computers) at least an hour before bedtime.

The blue light emitted by screens can interfere with the production of melatonin, a sleep-inducing hormone.

Mind Your Diet:

Avoid heavy meals, caffeine, and nicotine close to bedtime.

Opt for a light snack if hunger strikes before bed, and stay hydrated throughout the day.

Get Regular Exercise:

Engage in regular physical activity, but avoid vigorous exercise close to bedtime.

Exercise promotes better sleep quality and can help regulate sleep patterns.

Manage Stress and Anxiety:

Practice relaxation techniques such as deep breathing, meditation, or mindfulness to manage stress.

Consider journaling or creating a to-do list before bedtime to clear your mind.

Limit Naps:

If you need to nap, keep it short (20-30 minutes) and avoid napping late in the day.

Extended or late-afternoon naps can interfere with nighttime sleep.

Invest in Quality Sleepwear:

Choose comfortable sleepwear made from breathable materials.

Ensure your sleep environment promotes comfort and relaxation.

Seek Professional Help if Needed:

If sleep issues persist, consider seeking guidance from a healthcare professional or sleep specialist.

Addressing any underlying sleep disorders can significantly improve overall sleep quality.

Conclusion:

Smart sleep is not a luxury but a cornerstone of a productive and fulfilling life. By understanding the critical role sleep plays in physical and mental well-being, professionals can prioritize quality sleep as a proactive measure for success. Implementing practical strategies, such as establishing consistent sleep schedules, creating a relaxing bedtime routine, and optimizing the sleep environment, can transform sleep into a rejuvenating and empowering daily practice. As individuals embrace smart sleep habits, they lay the foundation for enhanced cognitive performance, increased efficiency, and overall well-being, setting the stage for a more productive and successful day.

Chapter 9

Navigating Social and Professional Networks with Grace: Building Meaningful Connections for Success

Introduction:

In the interconnected world we live in, the ability to navigate both social and professional networks with grace is a valuable skill that goes beyond mere networking. Building meaningful connections requires a delicate balance of authenticity, empathy, and effective communication. This article explores the importance of cultivating social and professional networks, the challenges associated with networking, and practical strategies to navigate these networks with grace, fostering genuine relationships and contributing to personal and professional success.

The Importance of Social and Professional Networks:

Opportunities for Growth:

Networks serve as a gateway to new opportunities, whether they be career advancements, collaborative projects, or personal development.

Well-nurtured networks provide a reservoir of resources, insights, and expertise that contribute to individual growth.

Knowledge Exchange:

Networking facilitates the exchange of knowledge and information.

Connecting with diverse individuals opens the door to different perspectives, fostering continuous learning and innovation.

Support System:

Networks can serve as a support system during challenging times.

Building strong connections enables individuals to seek advice, guidance, and encouragement from trusted peers and mentors.

Career Advancement:

Professional networks play a pivotal role in career development.

Job opportunities, mentorship, and career advice often come through professional connections.

Enhanced Visibility:

Being active in social and professional networks enhances one's visibility and reputation.

Positive interactions and contributions within these networks can lead to increased recognition and credibility.

Challenges Associated with Networking:

Authenticity vs. Image Management:

Balancing the desire to present oneself positively with the need for authenticity can be challenging.

Individuals may struggle to find a middle ground between showcasing their strengths and being genuine.

Navigating Power Dynamics:

Understanding and navigating power dynamics within networks can be complex.

Negotiating relationships with individuals of varying levels of influence requires finesse.

Building Meaningful Connections:

The quantity of connections should not overshadow the quality of relationships.

Building meaningful connections requires time, effort, and a genuine interest in others.

Overcoming Introversion:

For introverted individuals, networking events and social interactions can be draining.

Finding strategies to navigate networking situations comfortably is crucial for introverts.

Maintaining Balance:

Balancing the demands of a busy professional and social life can be challenging.

Individuals may struggle to invest time in nurturing relationships while juggling multiple responsibilities.

Practical Strategies for Navigating Networks with Grace:

Be Authentic:

Present your true self in both social and professional settings.

Authenticity builds trust and fosters genuine connections.

Active Listening:

Practice active listening to understand others' perspectives.

Engage in conversations with a genuine interest in what others have to say.

Find Common Ground:

Identify shared interests or experiences to establish common ground.

Shared connections create a foundation for meaningful relationships.

Effective Communication:

Develop effective communication skills, both in person and online.

Clear and respectful communication enhances your presence in networks.

Navigate Power Dynamics with Sensitivity:

Be aware of power dynamics within your network.

Approach relationships with humility, valuing every individual's contributions.

Cultivate a Diverse Network:

Seek connections with individuals from diverse backgrounds, industries, and experiences.

A diverse network provides a broader perspective and enriches your understanding.

Set Realistic Networking Goals:

Define specific and realistic networking goals.

Whether it's expanding your professional contacts or deepening existing relationships, setting clear goals guides your efforts.

Utilize Online Platforms Wisely:

Leverage social media and professional networking platforms strategically.

Curate an online presence that aligns with your professional goals and values.

Follow Up and Stay Connected:

After networking events or meetings, follow up with individuals to express gratitude or continue conversations.

Regularly check in with connections to maintain relationships over time.

Build a Support System:

Identify mentors, advisors, and peers who can serve as a support system.

A strong support network provides guidance and encouragement during challenging times.

Invest in Personal Development:

Invest in your personal and professional development.

Continuous learning enhances your value within networks and provides opportunities for collaboration.

Balance Quantity and Quality:

While expanding your network is valuable, prioritize the quality of connections.

Meaningful relationships contribute more to your growth than a large but superficial network.

Conclusion:

Navigating social and professional networks with grace is an art that combines authenticity, empathy, and effective communication. By recognizing the importance of building meaningful connections, understanding the challenges associated with networking, and implementing practical strategies, individuals can enhance their ability to create lasting relationships. In doing so, they not only contribute to their personal and professional success but also foster a network of support and collaboration that benefits the collective growth of the community. In the world of networking, grace becomes the guiding force that transforms connections into meaningful relationships and propels individuals toward success.

Chapter 10

Cultivating Joy: Finding Happiness in Everyday Moments

Introduction:

In the pursuit of a fulfilling and meaningful life, the quest for joy is a universal aspiration. Yet, joy is often mistakenly associated with grand achievements or momentous events. In reality, true happiness lies in the art of cultivating joy in everyday moments. This article explores the importance of finding joy in the ordinary, the psychological benefits of cultivating a joyful mindset, and practical strategies to infuse happiness into our daily lives.

The Significance of Finding Joy in Everyday Moments:

Gratitude and Appreciation:

Cultivating joy in everyday moments is synonymous with cultivating gratitude.

Focusing on the small, positive aspects of daily life fosters a sense of appreciation for the richness of our experiences.

Enhanced Mental Well-being:

Finding joy in the ordinary contributes to improved mental health.

Acknowledging and celebrating small victories and moments of happiness can reduce stress and enhance overall well-being.

Positive Perspective:

Cultivating joy is about adopting a positive perspective on life.

Embracing the joy in everyday moments shifts the focus from what's lacking to what's present, creating a more optimistic outlook.

Resilience in Adversity:

The ability to find joy in small moments serves as a buffer during challenging times.

Cultivating joy enhances resilience, helping individuals navigate difficulties with a more positive mindset.

Connection and Relationships:

Joyful individuals often create more meaningful and positive connections with others.

Sharing joy in everyday moments fosters a sense of camaraderie and strengthens relationships.

Psychological Benefits of Cultivating Joy:

Stress Reduction:

Finding joy in everyday moments has been linked to lower stress levels.

Positive emotions counteract the physiological effects of stress, promoting relaxation and overall well-being.

Improved Mood and Emotional Resilience:

Cultivating joy contributes to a more positive mood.

Individuals who regularly find joy in the ordinary tend to bounce back more quickly from negative experiences.

Increased Life Satisfaction:

A focus on everyday joy is associated with higher levels of life satisfaction.

The ability to derive happiness from small, routine activities contributes to an overall sense of fulfillment.

Boosted Creativity and Productivity:

Joyful moments are often linked to increased creativity and problem-solving skills.

A positive mindset enhances cognitive flexibility and can lead to improved productivity.

Better Physical Health:

Research suggests that positive emotions, including joy, contribute to better physical health.

The cultivation of joy is associated with lower blood pressure, improved immune function, and overall longevity.

Practical Strategies for Cultivating Joy in Everyday Moments:

Practice Mindfulness:

Be present in the moment and savor the simple pleasures of daily life.

Mindfulness allows individuals to fully experience and appreciate the joy inherent in ordinary activities.

Keep a Gratitude Journal:

Regularly jot down moments of joy and gratitude in a journal.

Reflecting on positive experiences reinforces the habit of finding joy in everyday life.

Celebrate Small Achievements:

Acknowledge and celebrate even the smallest accomplishments.

Recognizing achievements, no matter how minor, contributes to a sense of accomplishment and joy.

Create Rituals and Traditions:

Establish rituals that bring joy into daily routines.

Whether it's a morning ritual, a weekly tradition, or a bedtime routine, consistent practices create moments of joy.

Surround Yourself with Positivity:

Choose to spend time with individuals who bring positivity into your life.

Positive social connections contribute significantly to the cultivation of joy.

Engage in Hobbies:

Dedicate time to activities that bring genuine pleasure.

Engaging in hobbies provides an opportunity for joyous moments and creative expression.

Express Gratitude to Others:

Share your appreciation with others through compliments or expressions of gratitude.

Acts of kindness and appreciation contribute to a positive and joyful social environment.

Find Joy in Nature:

Spend time outdoors and appreciate the beauty of nature.

Connecting with the natural world often brings a sense of joy and tranquility.

Practice Positive Self-Talk:

Cultivate a positive inner dialogue.

Replace negative self-talk with affirmations and expressions of self-compassion.

Limit Screen Time:

Reduce time spent on electronic devices, especially on social media.

Excessive screen time can detract from the ability to be present and find joy in the real world.

Embrace the Power of Laughter:

Seek out opportunities for laughter and humor.

Laughter is a powerful tool for cultivating joy and improving overall mood.

Learn from Children:

Observe and adopt the joyous mindset of children.

Children often find joy in simple activities and can serve as a reminder to embrace the wonder and excitement in everyday moments.

Conclusion:

Cultivating joy in everyday moments is a transformative practice that transcends the ordinary and contributes to a more fulfilling and meaningful life. By recognizing the significance of finding joy in the small, daily experiences, individuals can unlock a myriad of psychological and emotional benefits. Through mindfulness, gratitude, positive social connections, and intentional practices, the pursuit of joy becomes a conscious and empowering choice. As we navigate the complexities of life, let us embrace the art of cultivating joy, finding happiness not just in grand moments but in the tapestry of our everyday lives.

www.ingramcontent.com/pod-product-compliance
Lightning Source LLC
Chambersburg PA
CBHW070751250726
48662CB00004B/1747